Naturally Beautiful
YOUR HAIR

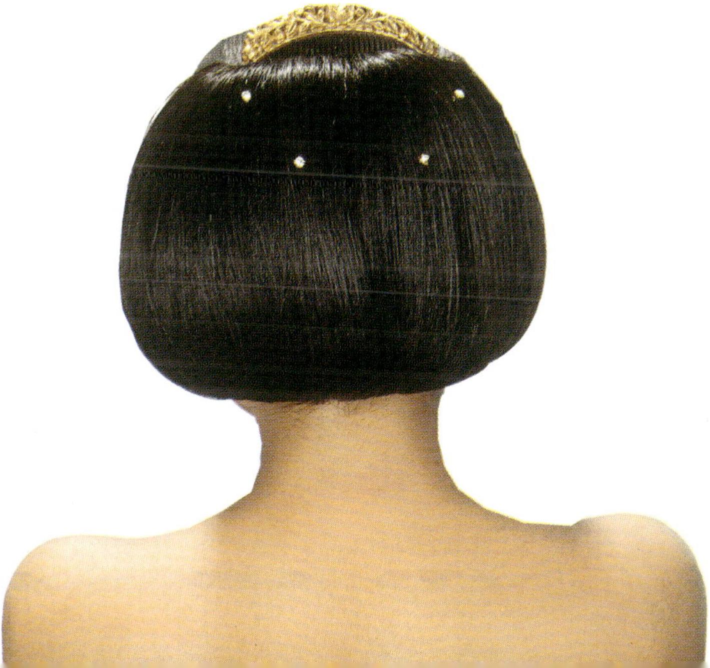

First Published 2002
Fifth Impression 2011

Published by
Rupa Publications India Pvt. Ltd.
7/16, Ansari Road, Daryaganj,
New Delhi 110 002

Sales Centres:

Allahabad Bengaluru Chennai
Hyderabad Jaipur Kathmandu
Kolkata Mumbai

Cover, Book Design, concept and styling: Peali Dutta Gupta
The Studio, S-94, Greater Kailash Part II
New Delhi 110 048

Printed in India by
Nutech Photolithographers
B-240, Okhla Industrial Area, Phase-I,
New Delhi 110 020, India

AMBIKA MANCHANDA

Naturally Beautiful
YOUR HAIR

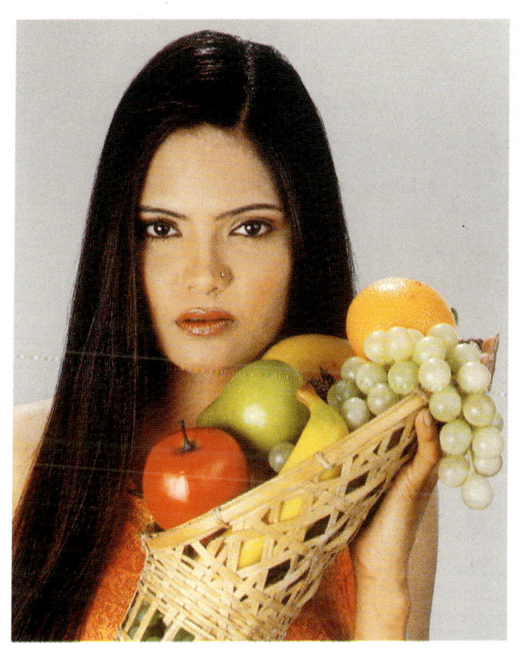

Rupa . Co

To my brother
Patanjali
and my father-in-law
Kailash

Sometimes you love because of circumstances.
And sometimes you love because of situations.
Sometimes you love no matter what.
And that is the best love there is.

Contents

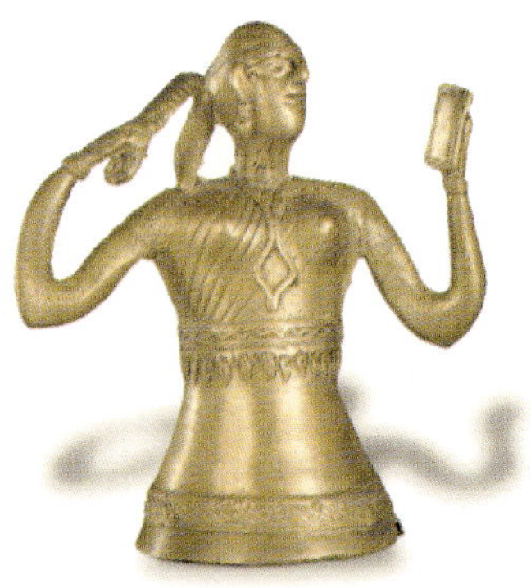

Foreword

Beauty is not the special shape of the eyebrows, the length of the hair, a tiny waist or dainty feet. It is more a way of expressing yourself, enhancing your physical assets and improving upon your drawbacks. Beauty is different things to different people. As the world changes, so do beauty concepts. How did black suddenly become beautiful? And lately, how is it that Indian women have taken all the top honours at the world beauty scene? Suddenly the world has woken up to the fact that beauty is not about looks, or colour, or about how to make up your face. It is much more than that. Its definitely about being comfortable with one's own body. Its about health and vitality. And most of all, its about the knowledge that I am beautiful, because I feel beautiful inside.

Being beautiful is all about lifestyle. Not the way society columns depict wannabes. Its about doing the right things, eating the right foods, and having a fitness and beauty regimen. To do the right things, one has to know what to do. This book takes a major step in that direction. It tells you how you too can be beautiful, with simple and effective directions. The remedies could well take you back on a nostalgia trip. We go back to nature and its bounty. It's a fresh look at grandma's recipes, and the kitchen. A plethora of beauty aids and treatments; easy to make and simple to use. And the results? Wait and see.

Oriental women from China and India as well as those from ancient Egypt were superbly skilled in the art of repairing the ravages of time. They made lavish use of flowers, herbs and resins for making applications and potions that made their skin glow. The ancient art of make-up, face care, and beautifying the body were far more elaborate and advanced than today.

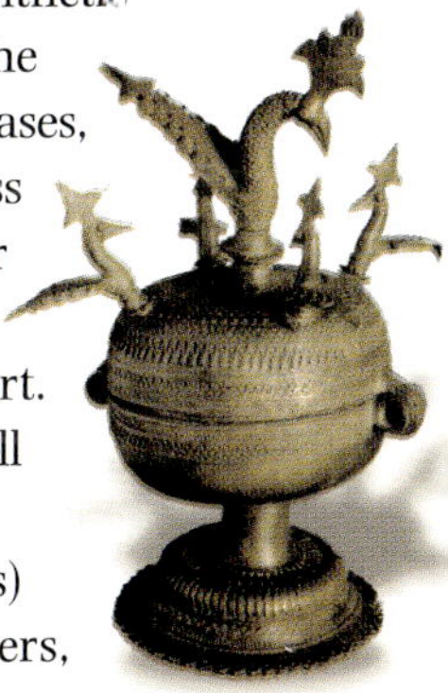

Shringar, or adornment, was considered almost a ritual for a bride. Traditionally and even today, at Hindu marriages the bride receive a beauty box from her husband. Today, synthetic mass manufactured vanity cases have replaced the ancient, adorably carved wooden chests or metal cases, once used by brides. Even the contents are mass products: a cream, a lipstick, a powder, and eyeliner and so on...as much as the purse permits. But in ancient times, the beauty box itself was a work of art. Much care was put into it and it was filled with all possible items for a woman's personal adornment. Glass or carved bottles of *attar* (extracts or perfumes) of roses, jasmine, mogra and many other flowers, containers of kohl for the eyes, others even more intricately carved or shaped containing *abeer* (powder) or *missi* (a herb) to redden the lips were lovingly put into the make-up chest.

Today women all over the world are using henna to disguise white hair and turn it to a reddish brown shade. In ancient times henna has been used not only to enliven the hair but also to adorn the palms of the hands and feet and even colour the nails.

Teenagers today, eagerly buy the latest anti-acne and anti-pimple creams at exorbitant prices, little realising that the cure for these ills exists in their own kitchens! Women in India have used sandalwood for centuries for this very purpose. It has strong antiseptic qualities and softens the skin. Similarly, women in most eastern countries have used "chikni mitti" or Fuller's earth, mixed with rose water. This is also popularly known as "Cleopatra's Pack" in the west. It helps to tighten the skin, and is the basis on which facemasks are marketed.

Women in ancient times were very particular about removing unwanted hair. Thus ash from incense sticks was used to get rid of them. Lemon juice and sugar mix was also used regularly for this purpose. Today, women go to beauty parlors for "waxing". Nothing changes. The future goes way back. Centuries back.

Women in India have always used herbs, fruits and flowers to beautify themselves, to adorn and enhance their good points. We do indeed have a wealth of knowledge as far as herbal and natural beauty aids are

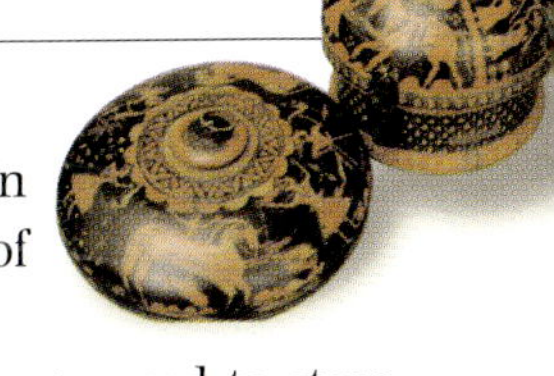

concerned. In fact beauty and make-up ritual in ancient times was more elaborate and state of the art than even today.

Exquisitely designed boxes and containers were used to store beauty aids. Historic evidence reveals that there was an intense desire for personal culture and body care. For instance, hair-drying pins of metal with intricately carved bases having devices for creating rhythmic sounds were used while drying the hair. These were very popular in South India. Among other objects of ancient toiletry articles, one can find slender bottles carved with tiny mirrors. *Kankavatis* were containers for a certain red pigment, used as bindis to mark the forehead. These containers had different forms like peacocks, musical instruments, elephants, swans, or were mango shaped.

Even the foot scrubbers found among ancient objects were imaginatively made. These also had a hollow shape and were fitted with tiny metal balls that made a rhythmic sound when used. Some other exquisitely shaped were containers for *Missi*, a herb to redden the lips; others contained different dyes to adorn the forehead. Carved boxes containing *Abeer* were also included. Abeer is a powder made from sandalwood, aloe, rose petals and a few grains of civet. These were powdered in a mortar to a very fine powder.

Thus the ancient art of makeup and adornment finds no comparison today. In this jet age of instant cures, we look backwards to the glorious days when it was difficult to find an ordinary face, when women made it a point to look extraordinary.

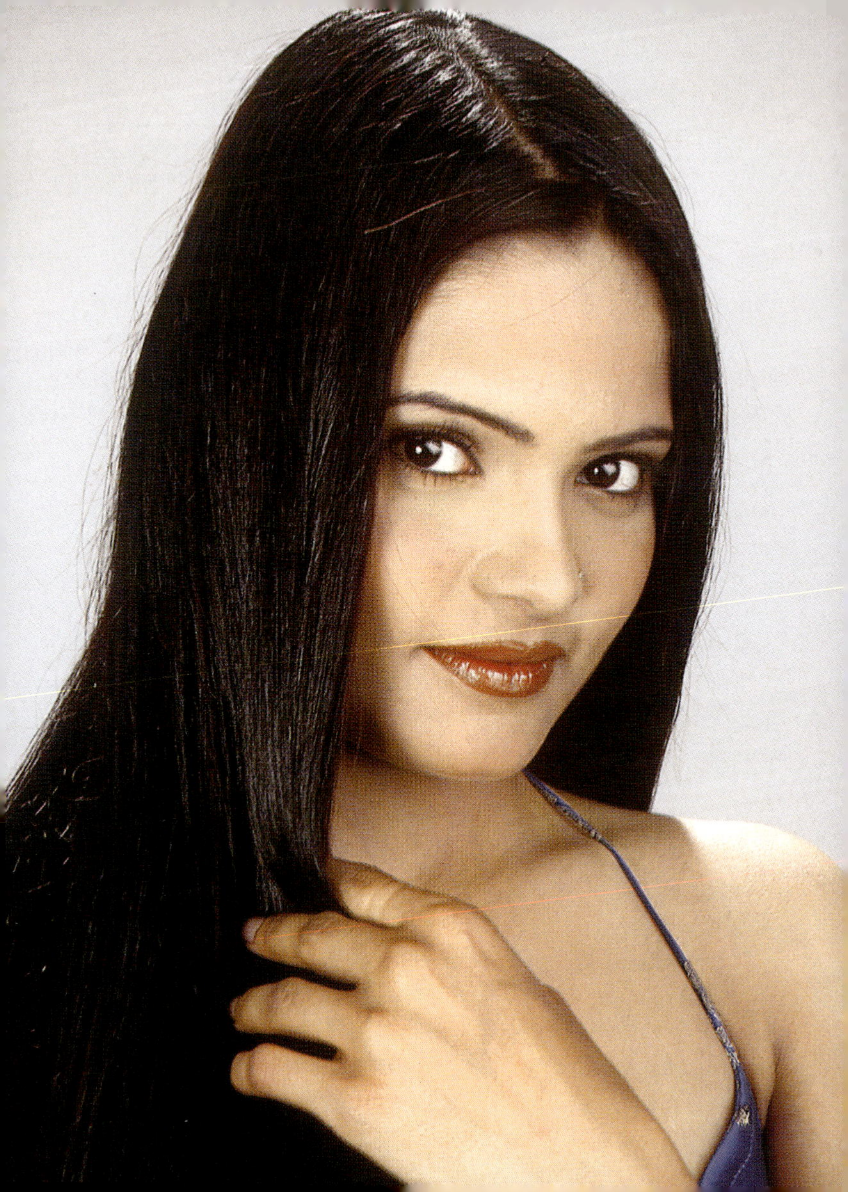

Your
Crowning Glory

Long, flowing, lustrous hair has always been associated with women of great beauty. Hair has also been an instrument of fashion, in fact it is often termed as a person's 'crowning glory'. Beautiful, bouncy hair reflects the health of a person; gives the appearance of vibrancy and life. Hair itself is organically dead material, but its follicles are not. The beauty and health of your hair depends upon the health of these follicles. Women spend fortunes on their hair. Well-groomed, luxuriant, lustrous, hair is, quite simply, beautiful and sexy. It can signify youth, health, and vitality.

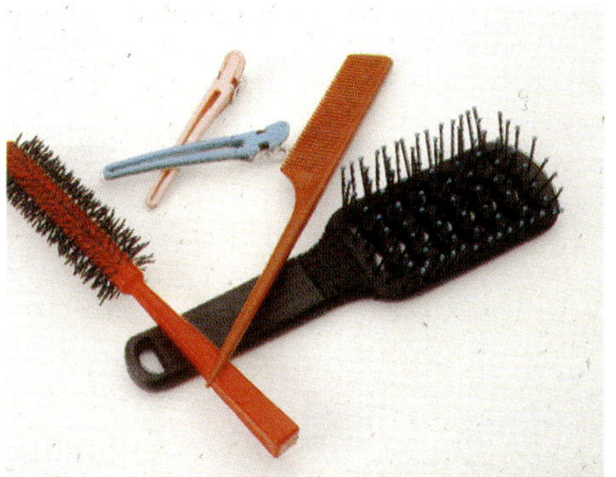

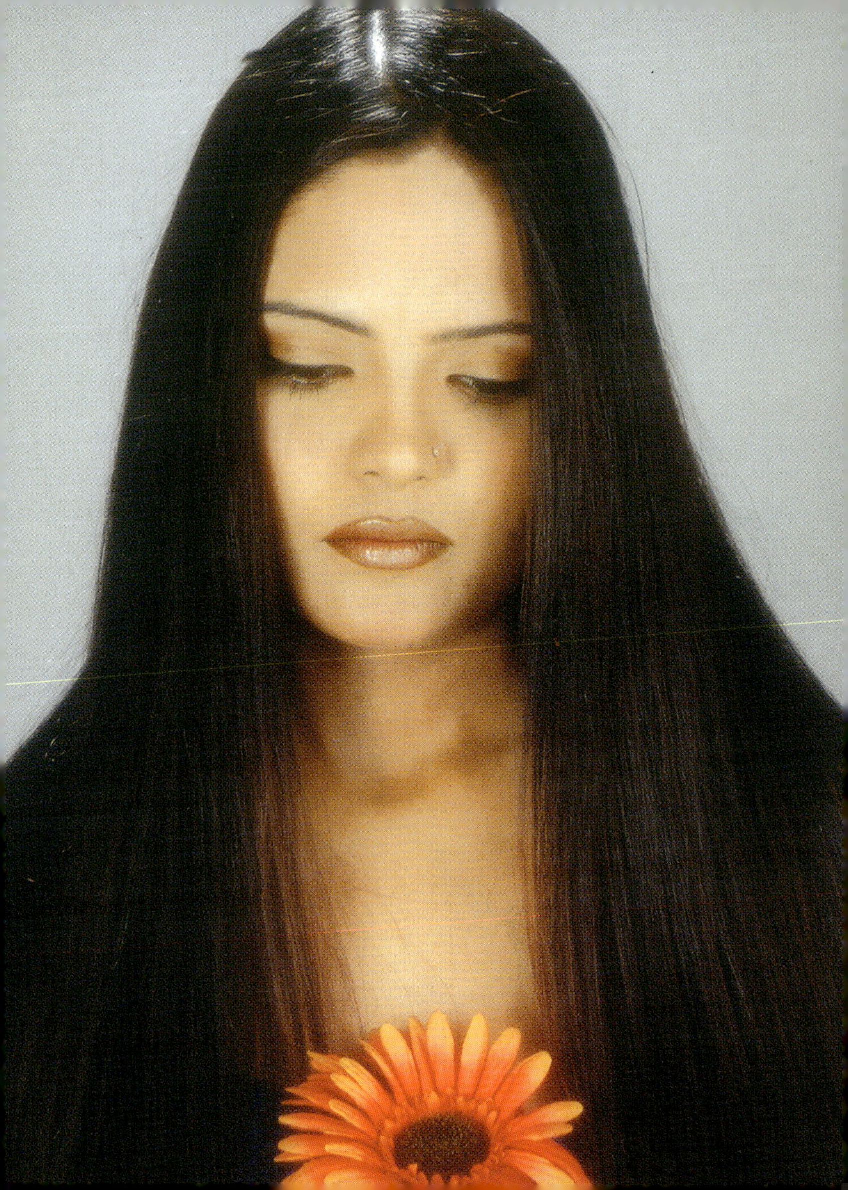

Hair goes through enormous "tortures" before it is made cosmetically acceptable to most women. Endless hours are spent combing, blow drying, tinting, curling, crimping, straightening, dying and bleaching. In fact, hair is subjected to endless experimentation. Indeed, it has amazing strength and resilience to cope with the vagaries of a woman's mind.

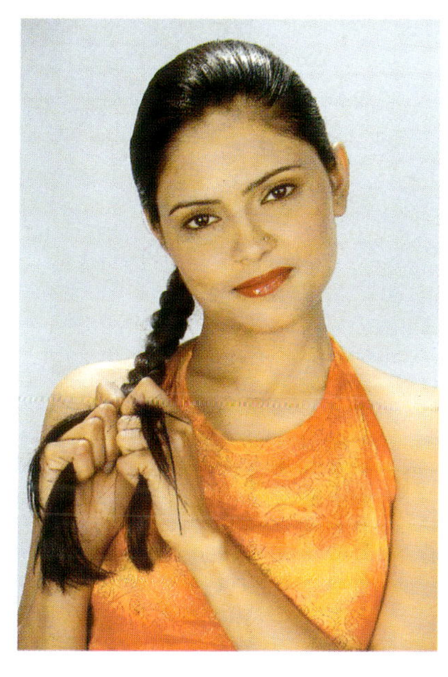

A woman's worst nightmare is loss of hair leading to baldness. Premature greying, rough and brittle hair are some of the numerous problems waiting to be solved. Hair comes in different textures, shades, colours, and is perhaps also a mark of distinction that differentiates between different races.

First, however, we need to know a few basic hair facts. Each hair is made up of an outer layer or cuticle. This is made up of a protein called Keratin, which protects the hair and helps retain moisture. Next is the inner layer where the colouring or pigmentation is produced. This surrounds the innermost layer, the medulla. Hair grows from a follicle on the scalp. Each follicle produces only one strand of hair. An average human head contains between 80,000 to 150,000 strands of hair.

A person's overall health is immediately reflected in the state of her/his hair. A healthy person sports thick, glossy hair. While baldness is usually more genetic in nature, a sudden loss of hair has a lot to do with external health factors. For women it could well be due to a reduced level of the hormone estrogen during pregnancy, hair loss due to anxiety and tension, hormonal imbalances, pollution, sudden weight loss, as also a badly mismanaged diet schedule.

The shape of the hair follicle determines your type of hair. Flat, oval shaped follicles promote curly hair, while perfectly round follicles promote straight hair. Hair colour is usually inherited and it complements the shade of the skin. Then, we have hair that is naturally dry or oily, fine or coarse, shiny or dull. There is a great variety.

Some of the most common problems are dandruff, split ends, thinning or falling hair, premature greying, dull and rough

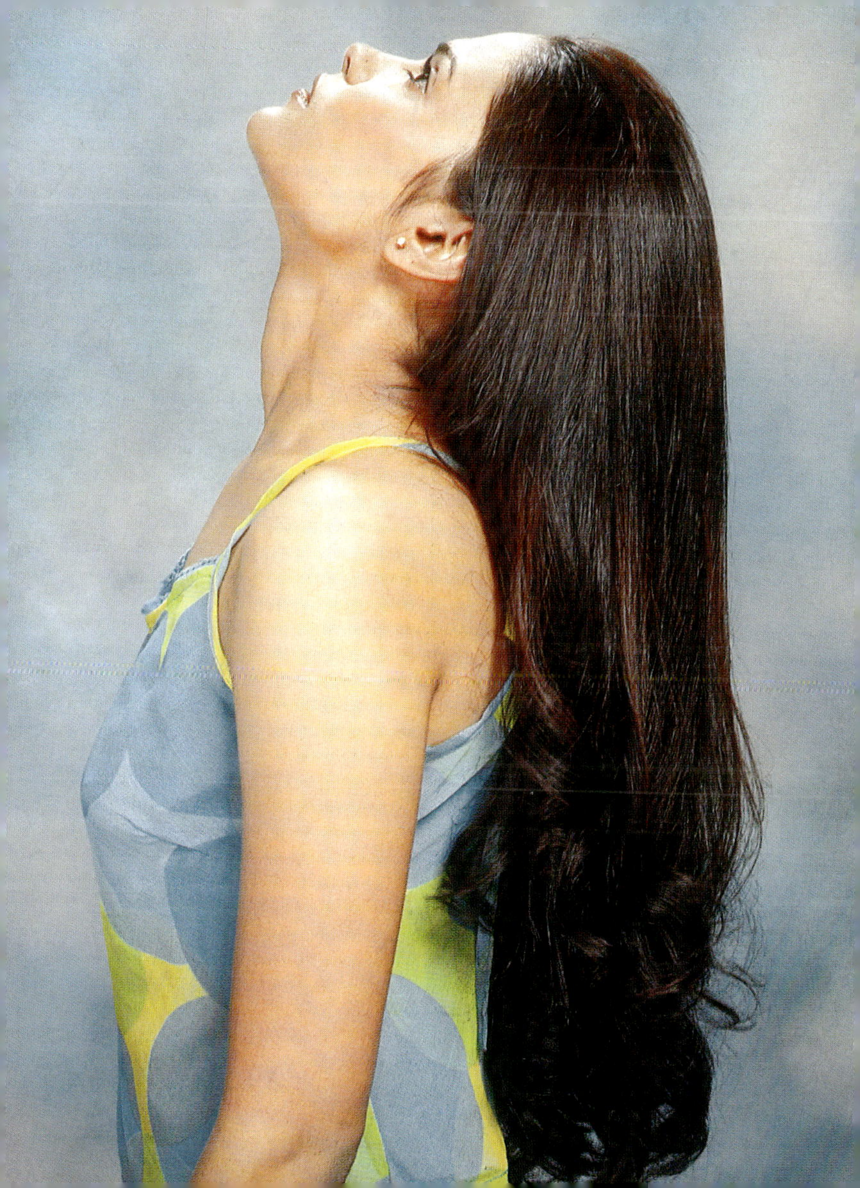

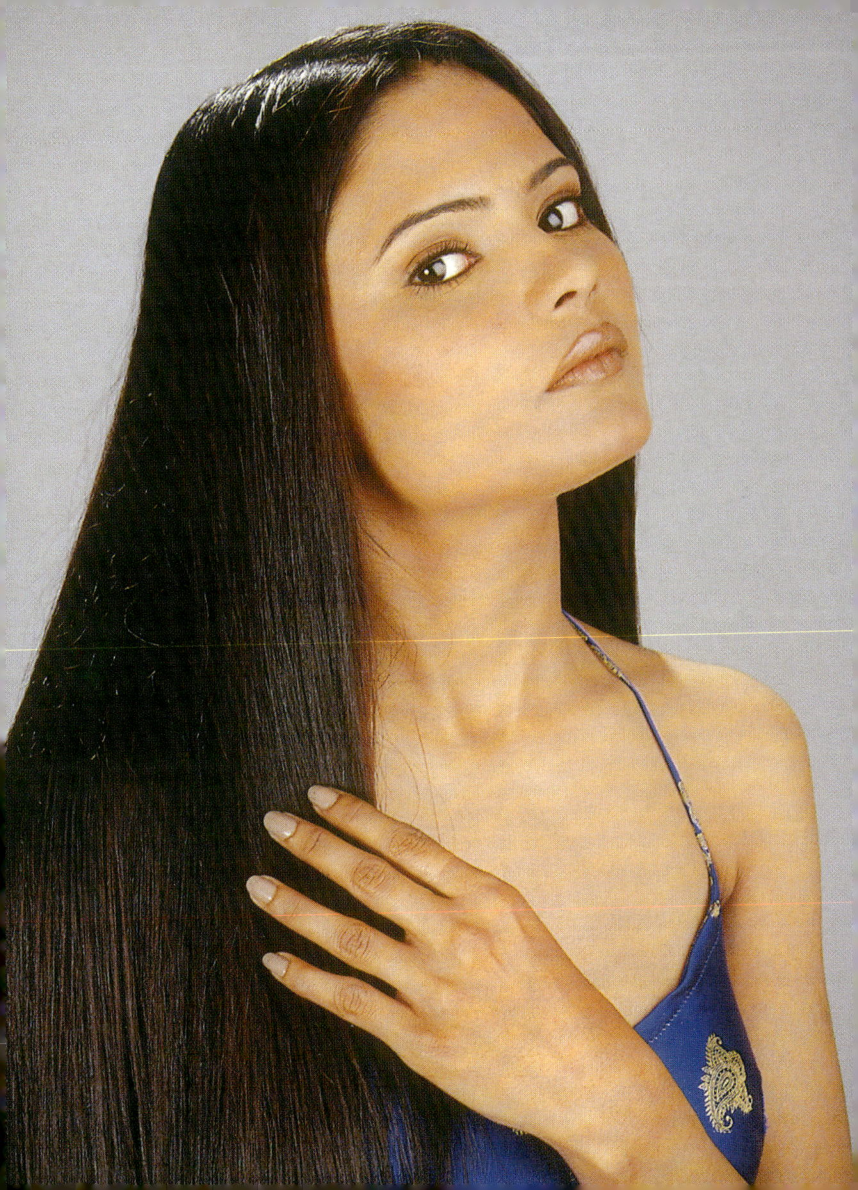

hair. Many, if not all of these problems can be tackled at home with natural products made from commonly available fruits, vegetables and herbs.

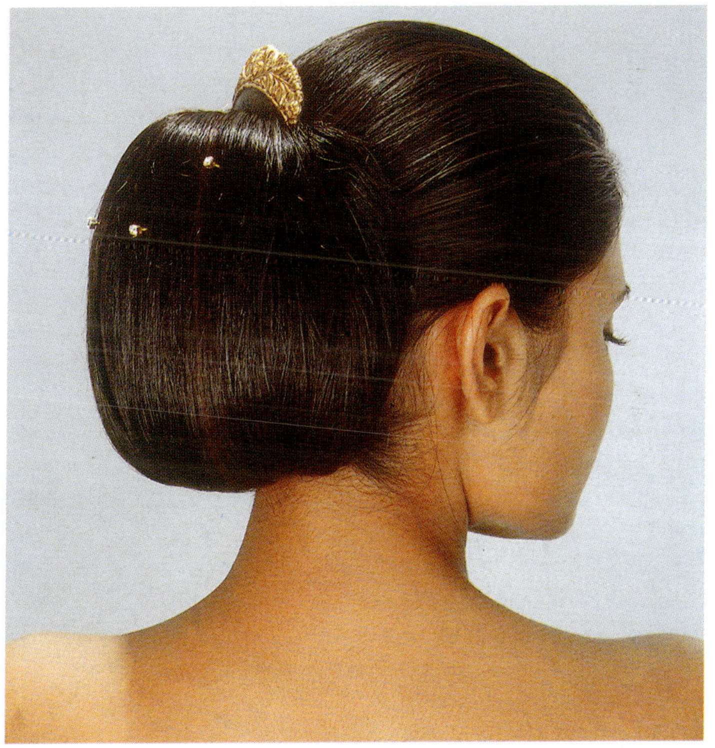

Dandruff

This is the most common complaint, and all of us suffer from this at some time or the other. There are a lot of misconceptions associated with dandruff. People who have this problem rush out and buy up the latest shampoos and conditioners.

There is also a misconception that dandruff is caused by dry scalp. In fact, it is due to an oily scalp. Wrong dietary habits like excessive consumption of cheese and chocolates also cause oil to accumulate on the scalp and cause dandruff. Worry and tension increase the flow of oil in the scalp, make you prone to dandruff. These white flakes can be a nightmare. Dandruff further tends to weaken the scalp, and the flakes falling on your face, neck and shoulders can affect your skin too.

WARM OIL TREATMENT: Warm 4-5 tablespoons full of wheat germ oil, olive oil or coconut oil. Massage well into the scalp. Wrap a warm towel around your head. Leave it on for 30 minutes. Rinse your hair thoroughly with water, to which lemon juice has been added. Massage well as you rinse. This is the most commonly known cure for dandruff.

CHICKPEA FLOUR (Besan) AND CURD: Take half a cup of chickpea flour. Add to this a little curd and enough water to make a thick paste. Apply on the scalp and individual strands of hair. Leave it on for 30 minutes. Rinse vigorously with warm water.

ROSEMARY AND OIL TREATMENT: Take half a cup of coconut or olive oil.

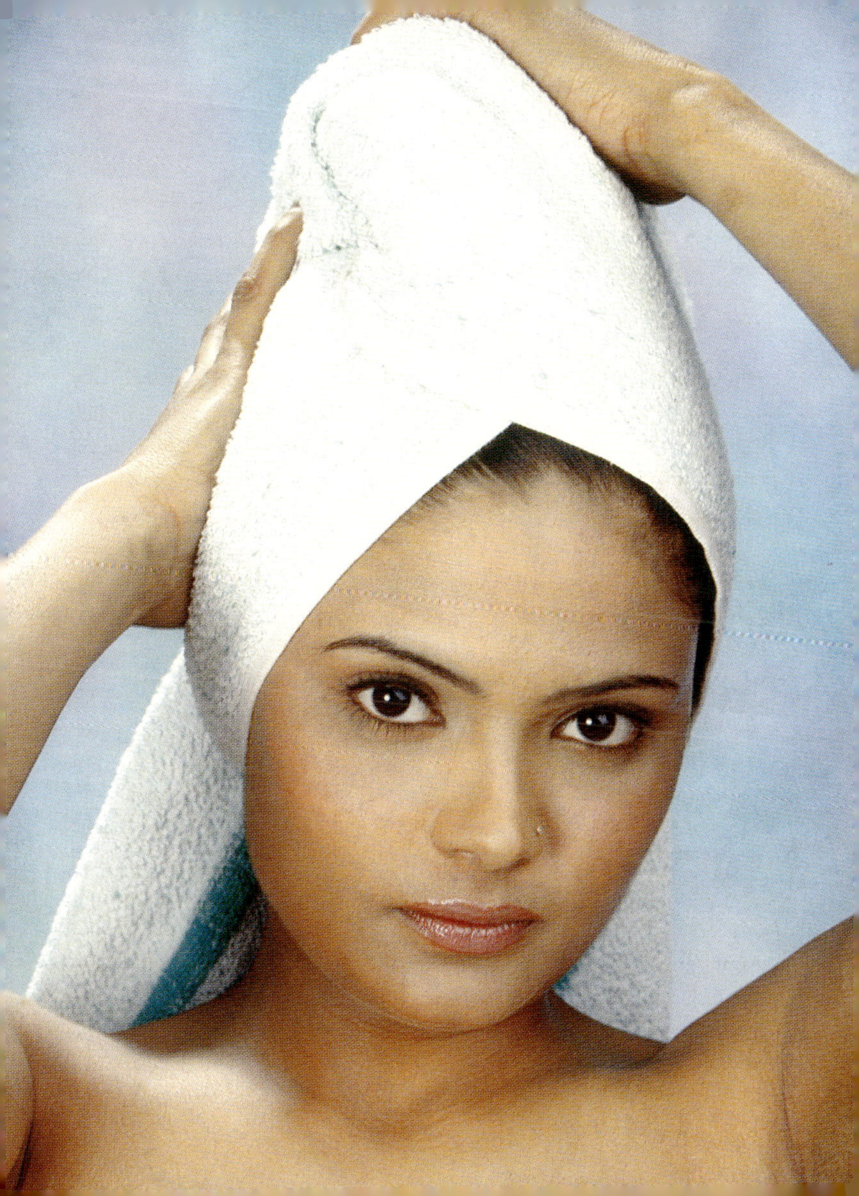

Add a few drops of rosemary oil, (alternatively, crush some fresh, or even dry rosemary leaves, boil them in the oil. Let it cool, then strain the oil by squeezing the leaves.) Apply all over the scalp. Leave it on all night after wrapping up your head with a towel. In the morning, rinse your hair with a mixture of warm water and lemon juice.

FENUGREEK (Methi) SEEDS AND OIL: Crush a tablespoon of fenugreek seeds in about 5 tablespoons of warm coconut or olive oil. It would be better to boil them in the oil. Cool the mixture and apply generously all over the scalp. Leave it on for two hours. Rinse and wash off.

SOAP NUT (Reetha): This is ideal for removing dandruff. Soak half cup soap nut overnight in one cup of warm water. Extract the juice from the soap nut by rubbing them vigorously. Strain. Apply directly on the scalp. Leave this on for 15 minutes. Rinse and wash your hair with tepid water. Shut your eyes tightly while rinsing as it hurts the eyes. Ensure that no residue is left behind.

ONION: Grind raw onions to a fine paste. Rub this paste into your scalp. Leave it on for an hour. Wash thoroughly. Rub in some lemon juice into your scalp and hair to rid your self of the onion smell.

BLACK PEPPER: Take 10 grams of black pepper powder. Add to it the juice of a fresh lime, along with a quarter cup of milk. Rub this mixture thoroughly into your scalp. Leave it on for an hour and wash it out thoroughly with water.

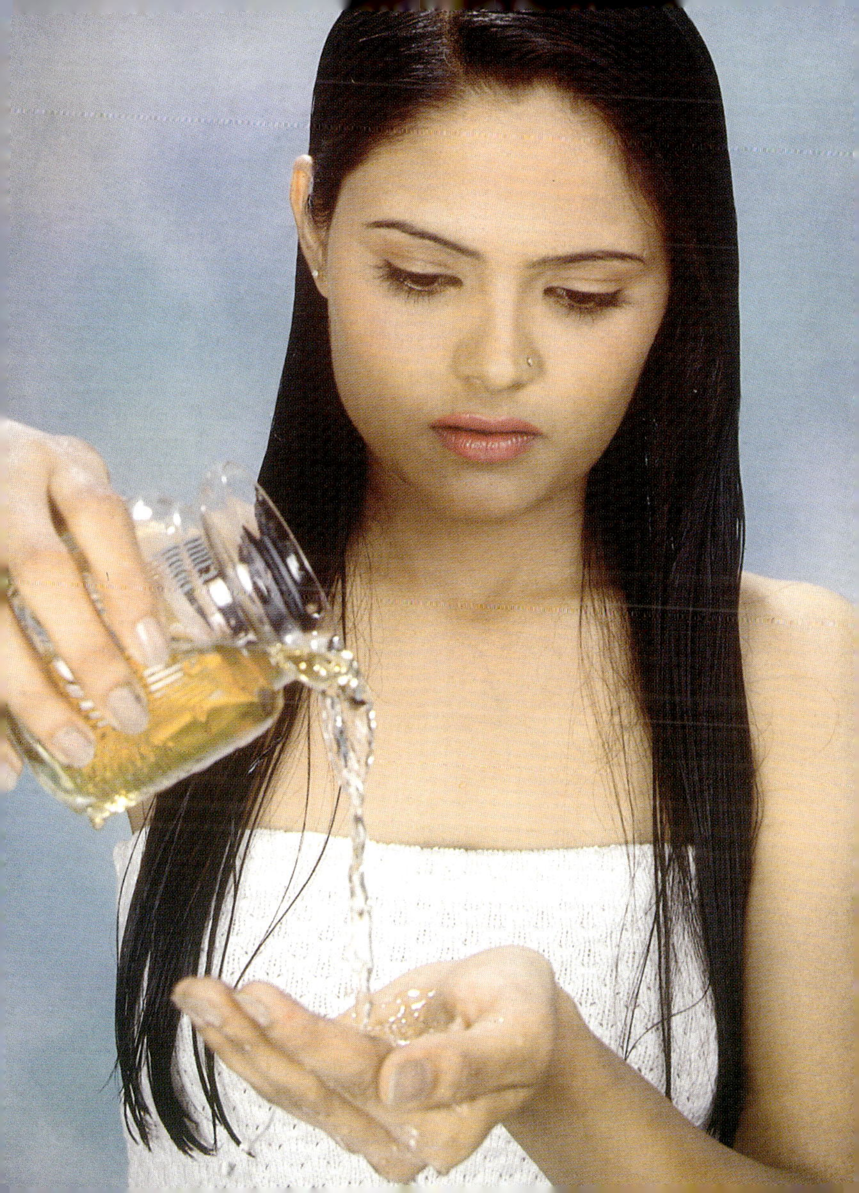

Dry Lifeless Hair

This hair looks like unwashed straw. It grows thicker nearer the scalp and thins out towards the ends, thus causing split ends. Atmospheric pollution too tends to have a drying effect on the hair. Such hair needs extra care.

WARM OIL MASSAGE: There is nothing as nourishing as a warm oil massage. Take half a cup of coconut oil. Crush 4 almonds and add to oil. Steam this mixture by placing it inside a pan. Apply while still warm, deep into the scalp and into the roots of your hair. Cover your head with a towel and leave it on for half an hour. Shampoo your hair.

BANANA NOURISHING PACK: Mash two ripe bananas. Add half cup beaten curd. Apply this paste all over your scalp and coat the ends of the hair with it. Pile up your hair high over your head. Leave it on for 15 minutes and then shampoo as usual. You will immediately notice a dramatic change in the texture of your hair.

EGG TONIC: Beat up an egg in a cup of milk. Squeeze in the juice of one lemon. Add to this a teaspoon of coconut oil or olive oil. Massage well into your hair. Cover with moist, warm towel. Leave it on for an hour. Rinse it thoroughly. The final rinse should be with lime juice and warm water. A good alternative would be to add yogurt instead of the milk.

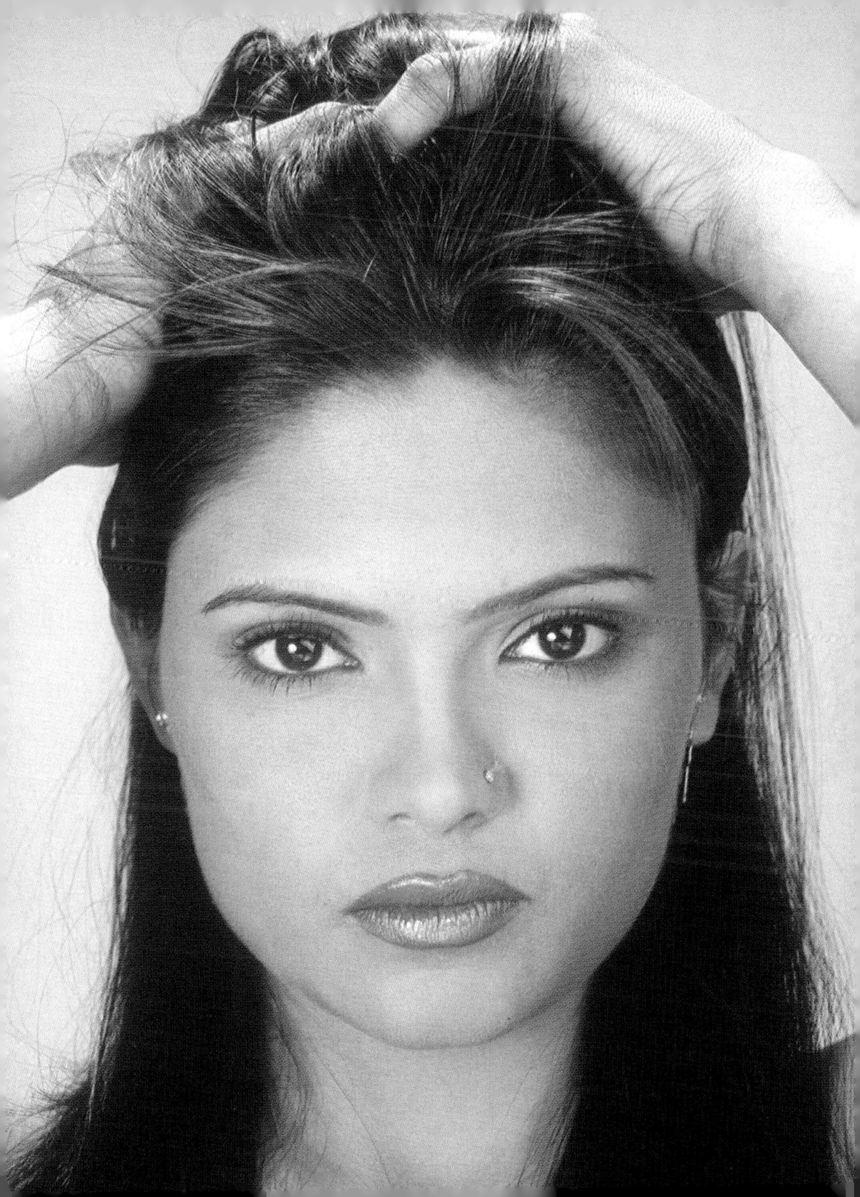

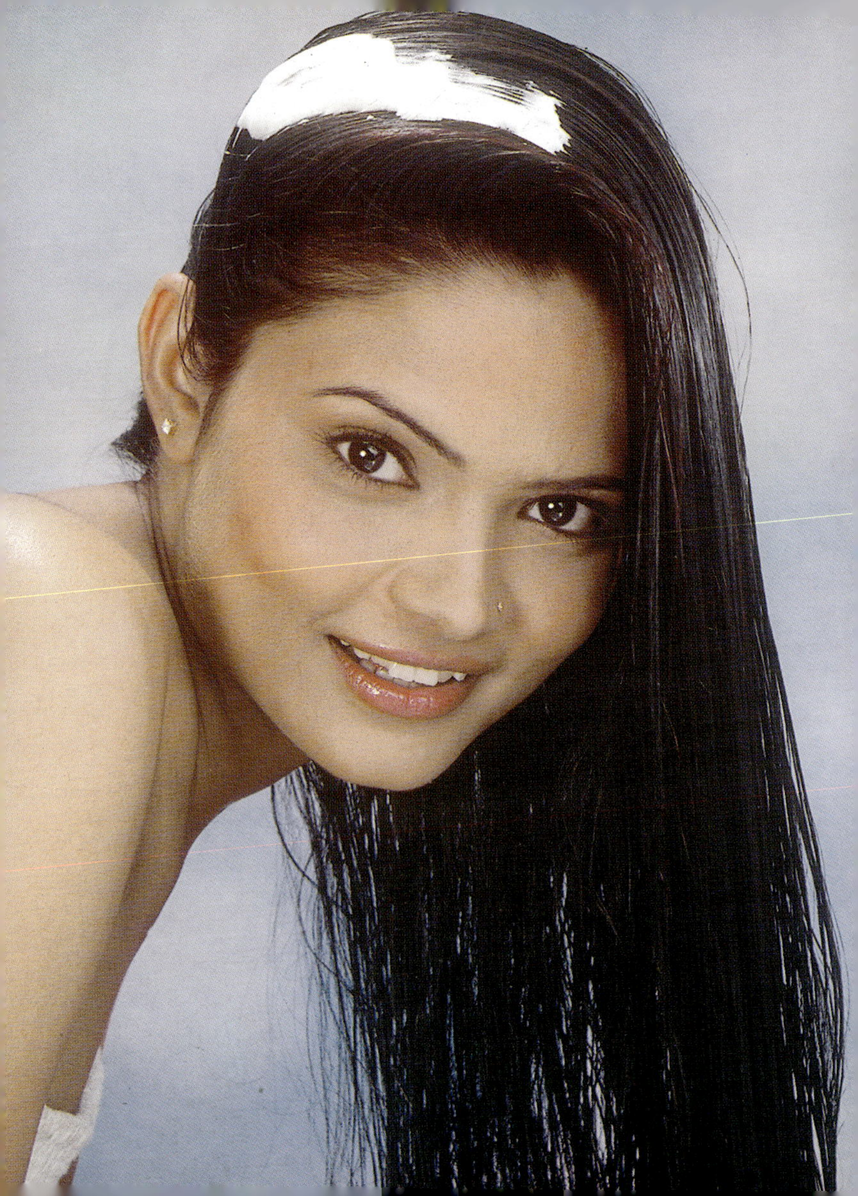

Split Ends

To treat split ends, first trim off the ends of your hair to an even length. Use all the nourishing applications described in the earlier chapter for your hair. Avoid back-combing or use of spiky rollers. You could also use these other nourishing tonic applications for your hair.

PAPAYA PACK: A unique, simple and easy remedy to bring your hair back to life. Take half of a ripe medium sized papaya. Slice after skinning and deseeding it. Put it in a blender and blend it to a pulp. Add half cup of yogurt and apply lavishly to your scalp. Part your hair at regular intervals and apply to hair strands and hair ends. Leave it on for 30 minutes. Rinse hair thoroughly with warm water.

CREAM TONIC: After you shampoo your hair, use the following tonic: take half cup milk; add to this a tablespoon of cream. Beat it up. Apply on scalp, hair strands and hair ends. Leave it on for 15 minutes. Rinse and wash well with water.

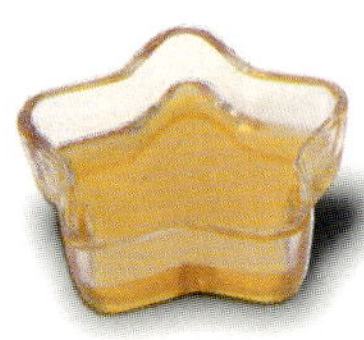

HONEY: Take half a cup of curd. Add to this a table spoon full of honey. Mix well. Apply on scalp and hair strands and hair ends. After 20 minutes wash with water. See a remarkable change in the sheen and smoothness of your hair.

BLACK LENTIL PACK: Take half a cup of black dal (lentil). Add one table spoon of fenugreek (methi) seeds. Dry grind to a coarse powder. Add half a cup of curd. Mix well. Apply generously all over the scalp. Leave it on for 2 hours. Wash your hair with water using a mild shampoo.

Any of these treatments should be a regular part of the attention that your hair deserves from you. The results? Seeing is believing.

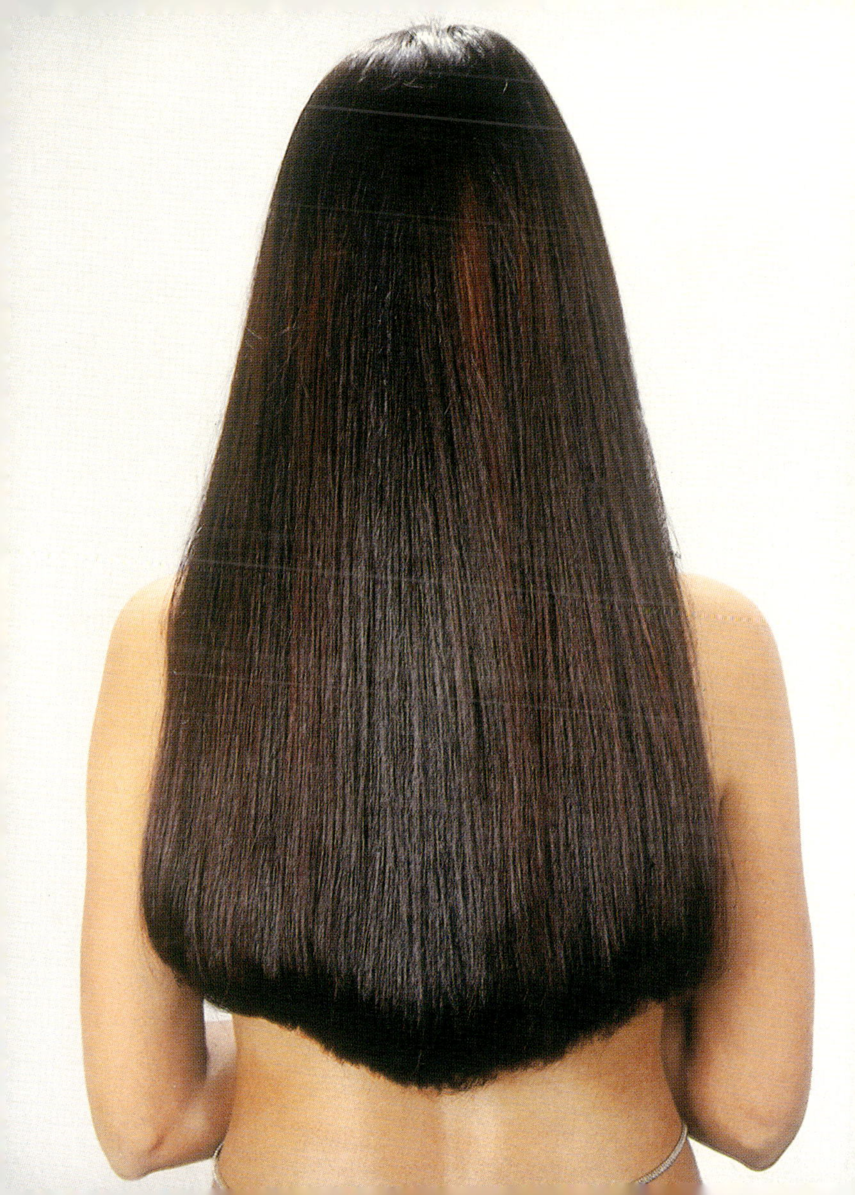

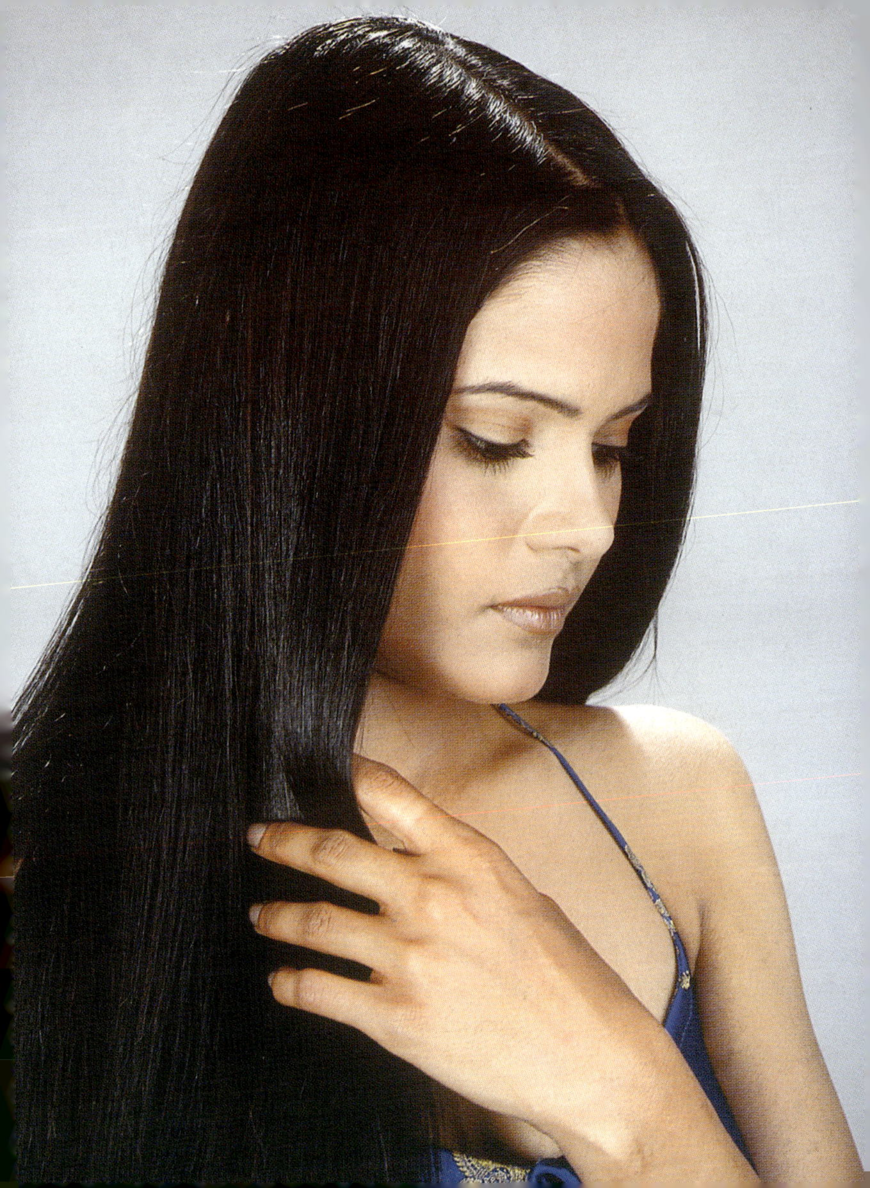

Greying Hair

The pigment Melanin controls the colouring of your hair. With advancing age, the quantity of pigment produced decreases, and your hair starts greying. Heredity too plays a major role in greying of hair. Pollution in the atmosphere and high chlorine content in water play havoc with your hair and cause premature greying. Natural treatment can arrest and delay this process. The watchword? Patience and continuity of treatment.

SAGE AND TEA APPLICATION: Put 2 tablespoons tea leaves and a handful of sage in a pan. Add half litre of water. Let it boil for 5 minutes. Cool sufficiently, strain the concoction and apply it to the roots of the hair. A very effective hair darkener.

HENNA: The universal favourite since the beginning of time. Used for colouring and covering grey hair. Acts as a tonic too, but has a drying effect; therefore best used along with a mixture of amla powder, boiled tea leaves in water and a little mustard oil. Apply this paste on your hair and leave it on for 2 hours. Wash off with water.

ONION PASTE: Few are aware of the magical properties of onion for your hair. Regular use of onion paste restores the original colour to your hair. Again, be patient and regular.

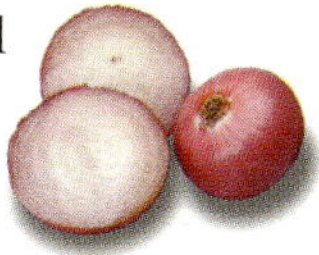

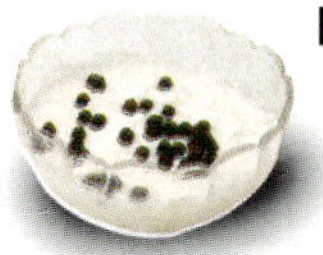

BLACK PEPPER AND CURD PACK: Take half cup curd. Add to this one table spoon of ground black pepper and the juice of one lemon. Apply this paste on your hair. Regular use helps in darkening your hair and the restoration of pigmentation.

WALNUT APPLICATION: Crush the fruit of the walnut and powder the outer shell. Boil in water. Strain and keep aside till it cools. Use generously and massage deep into your scalp. Leave it on for 20 minutes, then rinse with water. Helps in the retention of pigmentation of your hair.

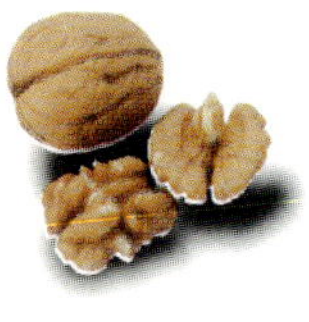

FENUGREEK (Methi) APPLICATION: Powder fenugreek seeds or chop fenugreek leaves very fine and boil in mustard oil. Cool, strain and then apply on your hair. Controls pigmentation loss.

AMLA, SHIKAKAI APPLICATION: Take 5 tablespoons of amla powder; 5 tablespoons of shikakai powder and 2 tablespoons of tea leaves. Put them on to boil. Pour the entire contents into an iron wok (karhai). Leave it overnight. The herbs absorb the iron from the wok and the mixture turns a deep black. Apply this thick paste all over your scalp, ensure that the strands and hair ends are also coated. Leave on for 30 minutes. Rinse and wash off with water.

BITTER GOURD (Karela) APPLICATION: Chop the bitter gourd along

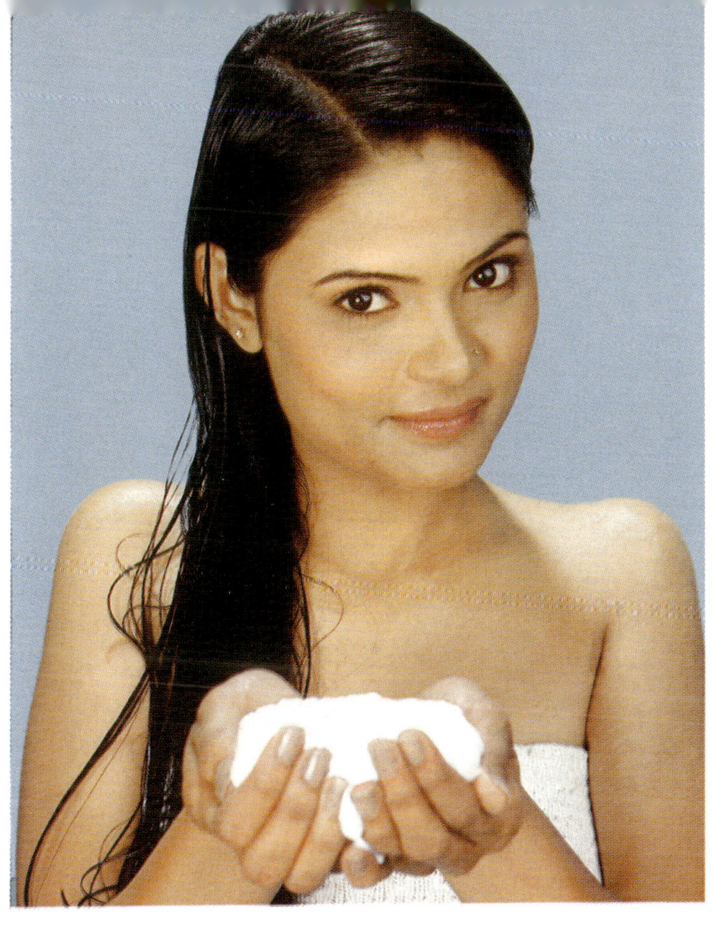

with the skin into thick round pieces. Soak in a bowl containing 1cup coconut oil. Leave it for 4 days. Boil, cool and strain after squeezing the bitter gourd juice into the oil. Use this oil regularly. Helps in darkening the hair and restoration of pigmentation.

Oily Hair

This type of hair is very fine in texture. It is easily affected by atmospheric pollution and needs to be shampooed and washed more often. If you have oily hair, then try and keep it covered when going out in the sun. Diet too is important. Avoid fried foods and dairy products. Increase your intake of fresh fruits, green and leafy vegetables and salads. Drink plenty of water.

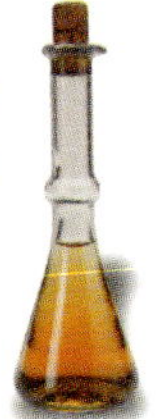

LIME AND VINEGAR RINSE: Take a cup of warm water and add three tablespoons of vinegar along with the juice of one lemon. Gently massage this mixture into your hair and scalp. Leave it on for 30 minutes. Wash and rinse with water.

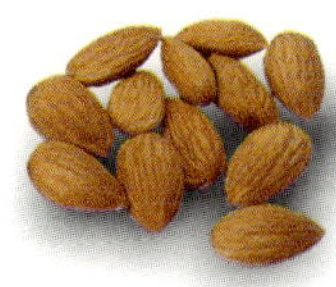

ALMOND OIL AND WATER APPLICATION: Take half cup water, add to this a teaspoonful of almond oil. Massage this into your hair half an hour prior to your bath. Shampoo and rinse off. Note, the massage is with oil and water emulsion. Do not use only the oil.

BAKING SODA RINSE: The hair accumulates dirt very quickly. In addition, there is a build up of shampoo and conditioner. It alters the alkaline (pH) levels, making the hair oily and limp. Here is a quick rejuvenation application. Take a tablespoon of baking soda, add to it 4 tablespoons of cider vinegar. Rub this into your scalp, leave it on for 5-7 minutes and shampoo your hair. It comes out

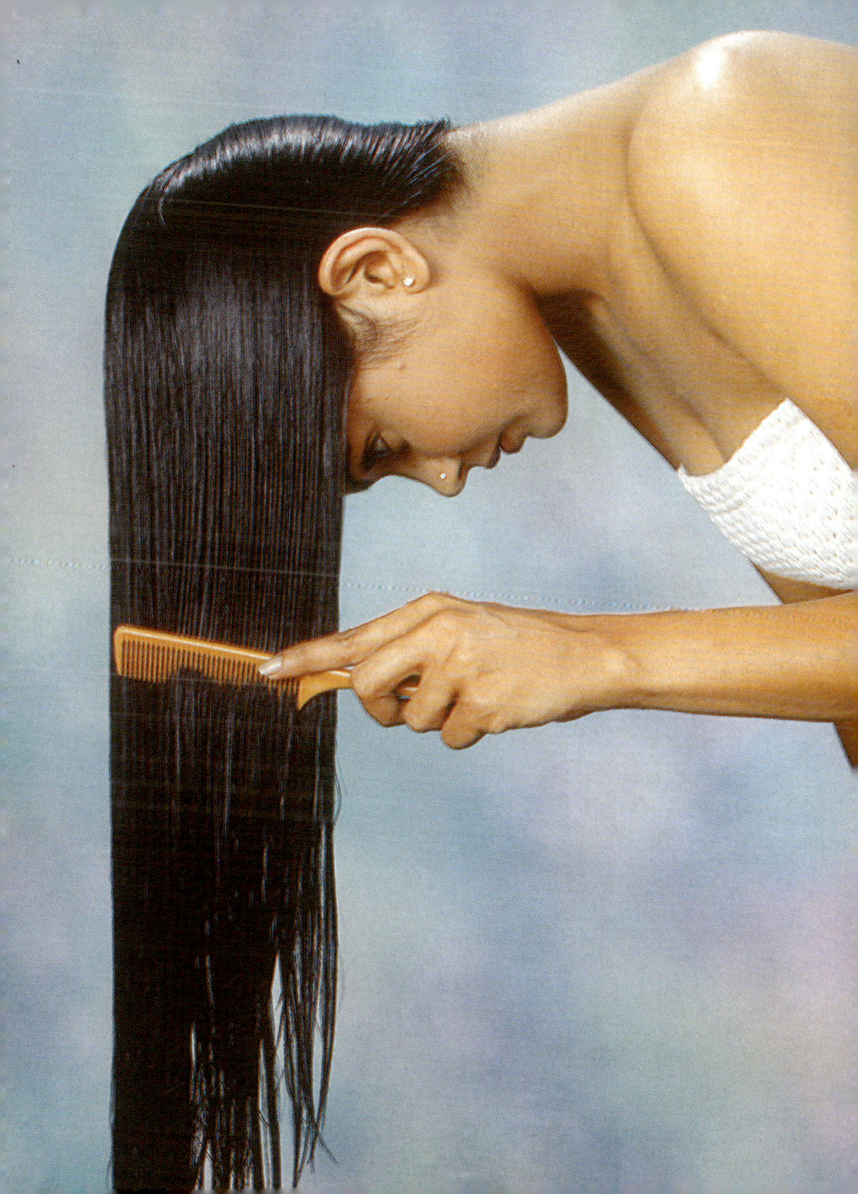

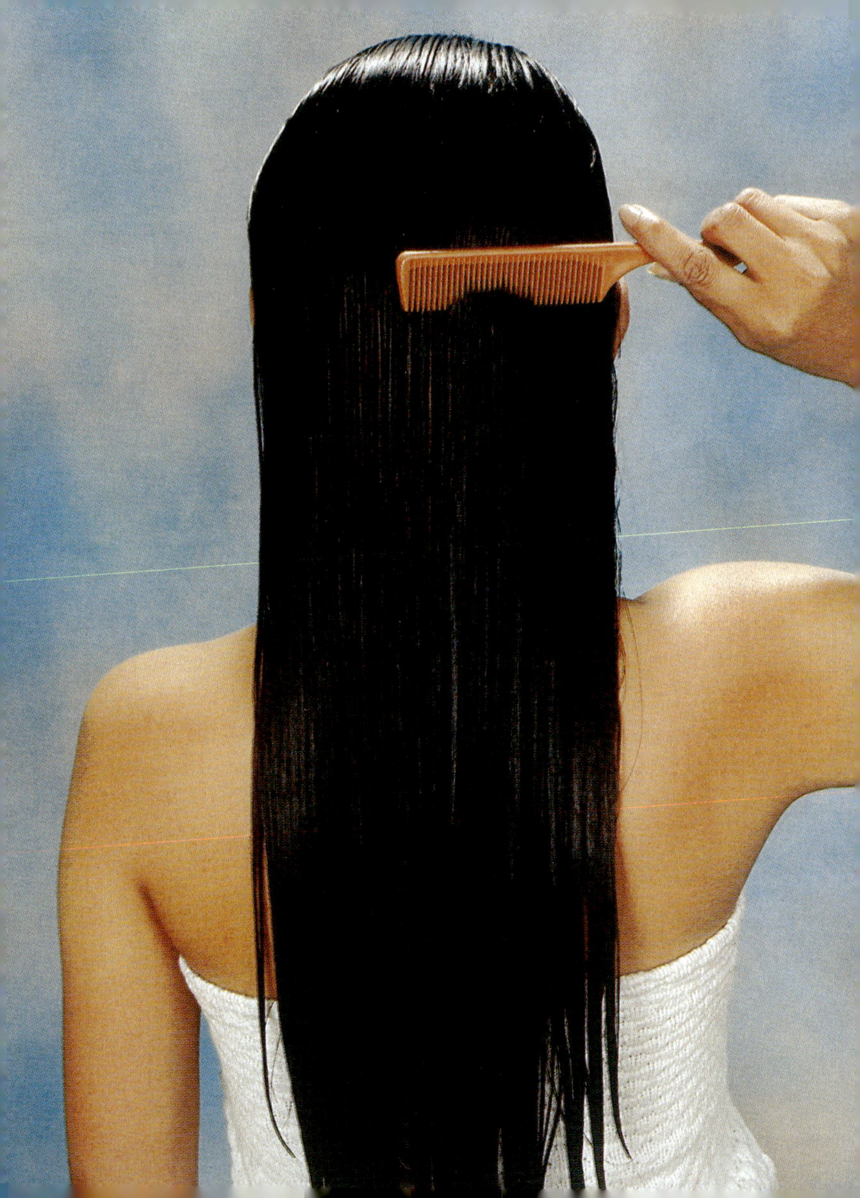

squeaky clean, vivacious and buoyant.

COLOGNE RUB: Mix equal parts of any cologne and water. Use cotton wool to rub this mixture into fine partings of the hair. This lifts grease of the roots. Wash hair as usual.

APPLE AND VINEGAR RINSE: Grate one apple. Add to it half cup vinegar. Apply generously all over scalp and length of hair. Leave it on for 20 minutes, wash off, rinse thoroughly.

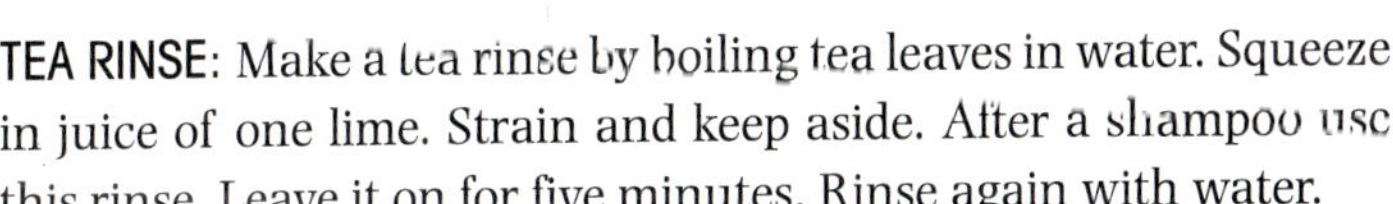

TEA RINSE: Make a tea rinse by boiling tea leaves in water. Squeeze in juice of one lime. Strain and keep aside. After a shampoo use this rinse. Leave it on for five minutes. Rinse again with water.

Homemade Hair Conditioners

Fruits, vegetables and even nourishing food are miraculous hair conditioners if used in the right way.

AVOCADO: Chop and put fruit in blender. Mix 2 egg yolks in this pulp. Massage well into hair. Rinse with a mixture of lime juice and vinegar.

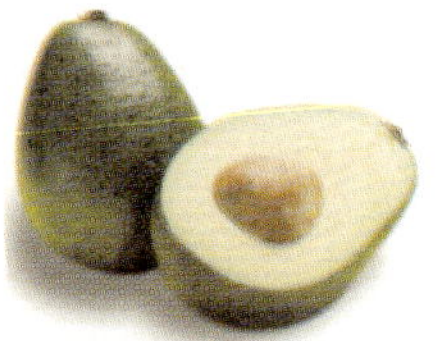

MAYONNAISE: Food for hair! Heat half cup of mayonnaise. Apply to dry, unwashed hair. Leave it on for half an hour. Rinse, then shampoo. Gives super results.

SAFFRON: Boil saffron strands in water. Cool it. Add to it the juice of one lime and one tablespoon of honey. Rub into scalp and hair strands. Leave it on for 15 minutes. Rinse thoroughly with water. Your hair acquires a golden sheen.

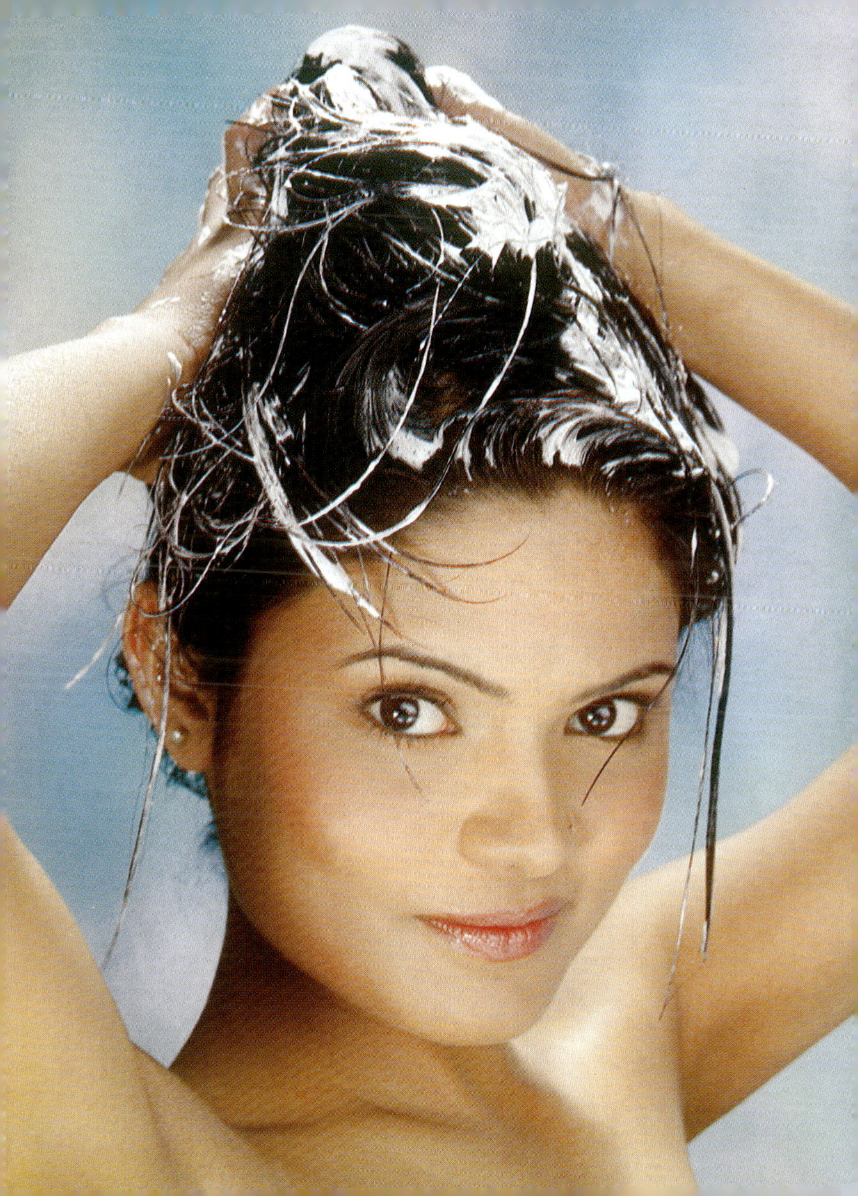

Helpful Tips

Some people are genetically prone to grey hair, thinning hair or balding. However, the health of your hair depends largely on your blood circulation and nutrition. Without adequate protein inputs in our body, hair stops growing. Its colour changes and it becomes brittle and lifeless. Thus, ensure that you have protein with foods.

Sometimes low hemoglobin results in hair loss. This is due to iron deficiency, which can be overcome by eating bananas, apples and other iron enriched foods.

Avoid eating refined foods like chocolates, burgers, pizzas and pastries. Yeast tablets help hair growth, so does Vitamin E. Other foods that promote hair growth are grains, beans, lentils, green leafy vegetables particularly fenugreek, carrot juice, beetroot juice, fish and fruits like avocado, apple and banana. Here are a few tips for your crowning glory.

- A regular hair care regime should be followed.
- Tie a scarf if you are going out in the hot sun. A hundred strokes at night as granny advised should not be forgotten. Brush firmly, but not harshly, by putting your head forward and throwing your hair in front. Brush neck downwards and outwards.
- A warm oil massage regularly is a must.
- Be careful when using a conditioner, avoid using it on the scalp, only on the hair strands.
- Do not apply the shampoo directly onto the hair. Take a little water in the palm of your hand and mix the shampoo first

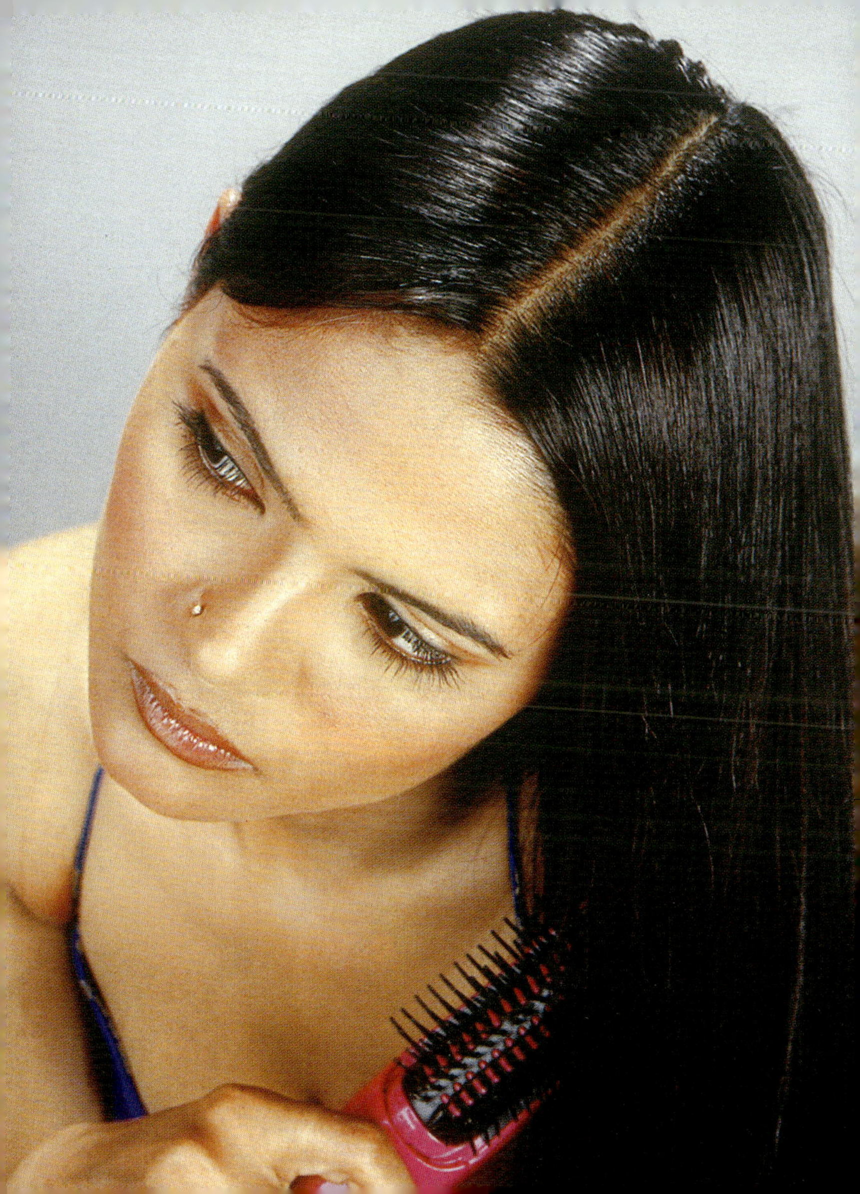

before applying on the hair.

- After shampooing your hair, it is always better to rinse the hair too.
- Occasionally rinse your hair with some of the rinses mentioned above.
- Choose the right kind of brush for your hair. Flat brushes are best for normal use. Use round and vented brushes for blow drying, while a cushioned brush body is best because it moulds itself to your contours.
- Always ensure that you follow a regular cleaning and nourishing routine.
- So it is about going back to the basics. It is about healthy hair, and feeling good with a little help from nature.

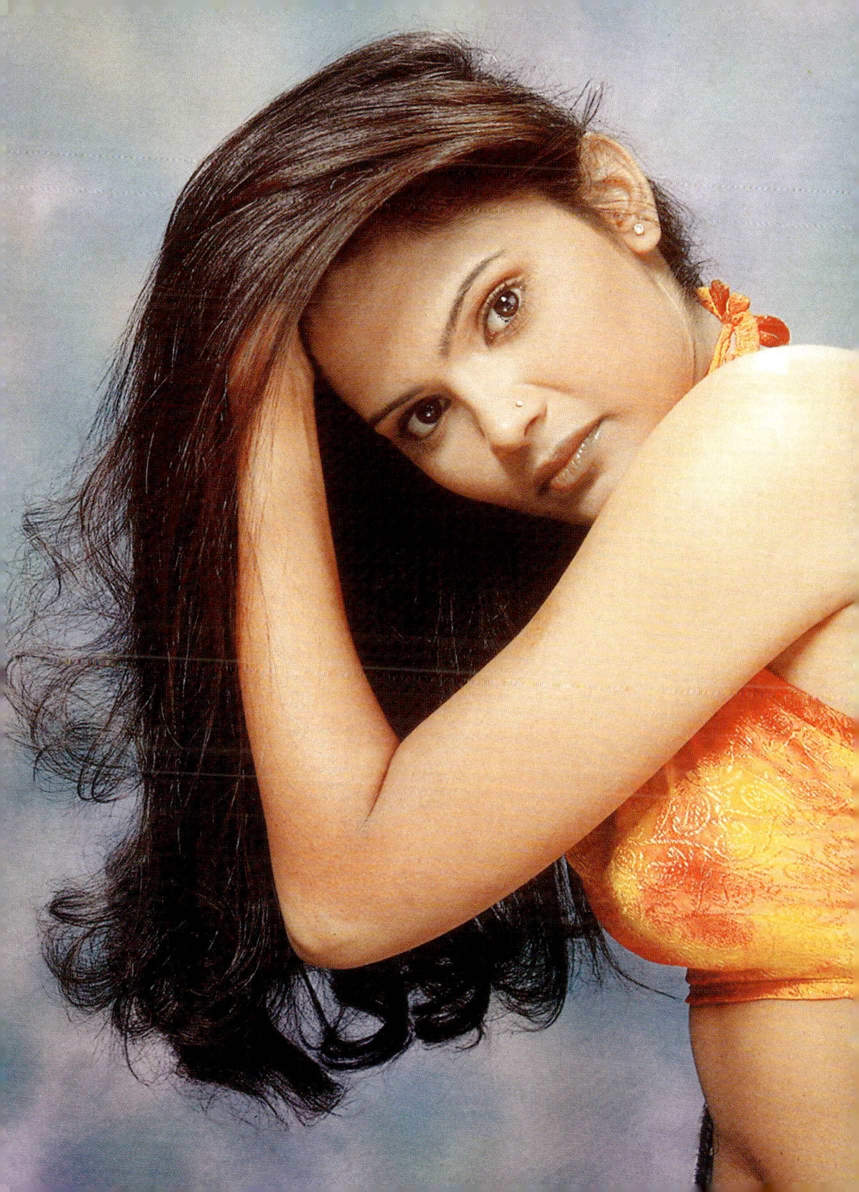

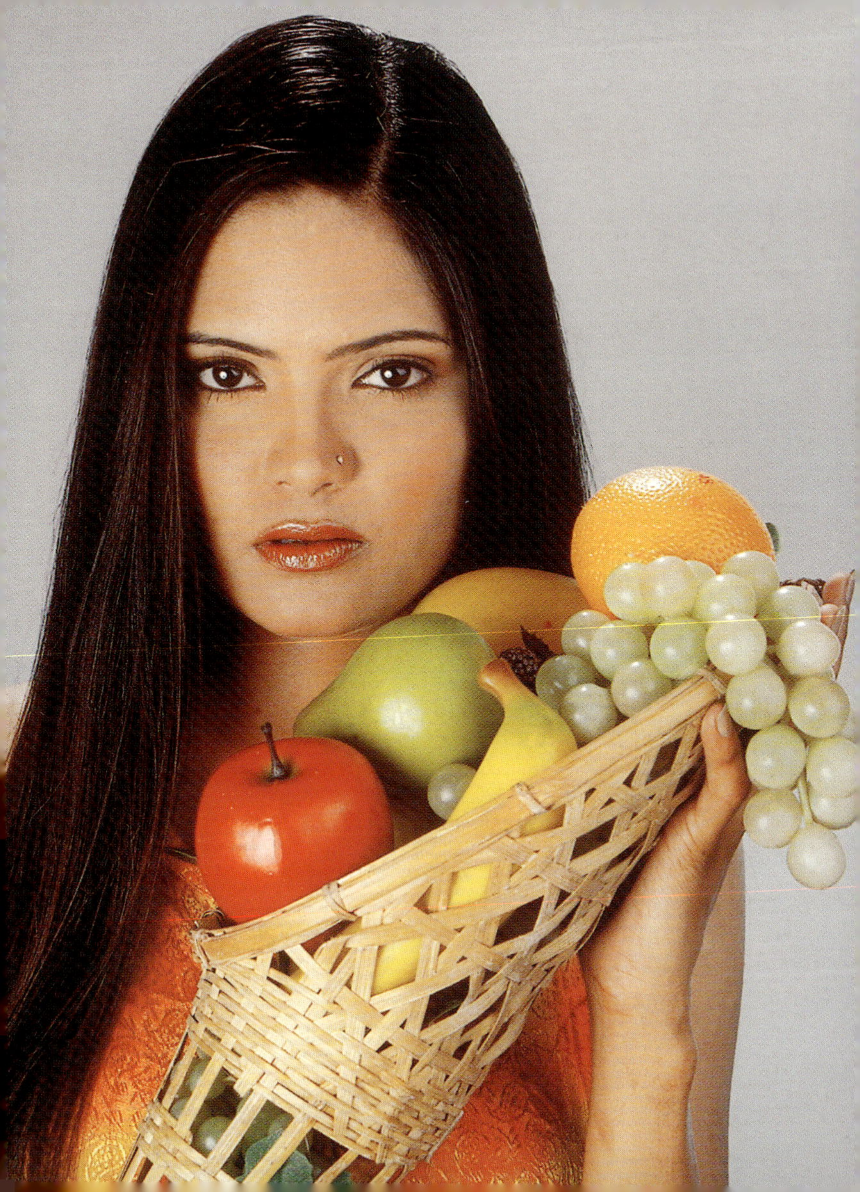

Eat and Grow Beautiful

Looking beautiful and retaining one's beauty should not make you an obsessive slave to beauty cures. While the right use of make-up and beauty care products can undoubtedly enhance your beauty, you can be truly beautiful only if you are healthy. So, eat the right food and grow beautiful. Once you gain knowledge about the right kinds of foods for good health, you can start eating a well-regulated diet, and the results will only be too evident. Your face will glow with health and vitality, your hair will bounce and shine, and your body will be taut and trim. It makes a lot of sense to care not only about the food you eat, but also in the manner in which you do so. A few tips on practical knowledge about food and eating habits would certainly go a long way into developing a healthy regime, which will stand you in good stead.

Undoubtedly, beauty is also a state of the mind. In order to look good, you ought to "feel good" too. True beauty comes from within, from a feeling of well-being. It is not the way you dress, or do your make-up, nor your sense of style or get up, but it is the person within you that looks radiant and beautiful.

Good looks have a lot more to do with food than is commonly realised. The key to vitality, health and beauty is in eating right.

Women in general, and working women in particular, ignore their basic food requirements, leading to malnourishment and other deficiencies. Today, in any urban environment, as much as 75% of young working women are anaemic. This also results in period cramps, heavy bleeding, abdominal bloating and irritability. All this takes a heavy toll on your body and in the way you look. Coupled with this is the fact that many urban women are prone to emotional dieting fads, which messes up the delicate balance within the body, and deprive themselves of essentials like iron, calcium, proteins and minerals. Eventually, this affects the hair, skin, and teeth, and gives the appearance of premature ageing. Bulimia and Anorexia are also growing as women look to magazines and glossy ads and try to be like the thin emasculated models that promote the business of beauty.

Excess of carbohydrates for instance, can take a toll on the hair, skin and the eyes. On the flip side, the addition of vitamins and other nutrients to food can make a difference in the quality of your skin, your hair, and remove headaches and irritability and other day-to-day ailments. Did you know that sluggishness and lack of energy could be overcome with a changed and improved diet plan?

All this does not imply that you need to be fastidious or obsessive about your food. It only means that you need to have basic nutritional awareness about your food. You can thus select the right kinds of foods best suited to the needs of your body. Its your daily food intake that is important. So, do spare a thought for food. Make sure that you get enough nutrients and have a balanced diet. This is the key to good health and beauty. Modern day eating habits, convenient cooking and fast food culture robs us of essentials like vitamin B complex, as found in milk, liver, fish and wheat germ. We tend to cultivate wrong eating habits. Let me just tell you very briefly about some nutrients that are absolutely essential for a sound and healthy body.

Skin: Your skin needs Vitamin B2. This is present in fresh vegetables, milk, whole wheat bread. It also needs Vitamin C to

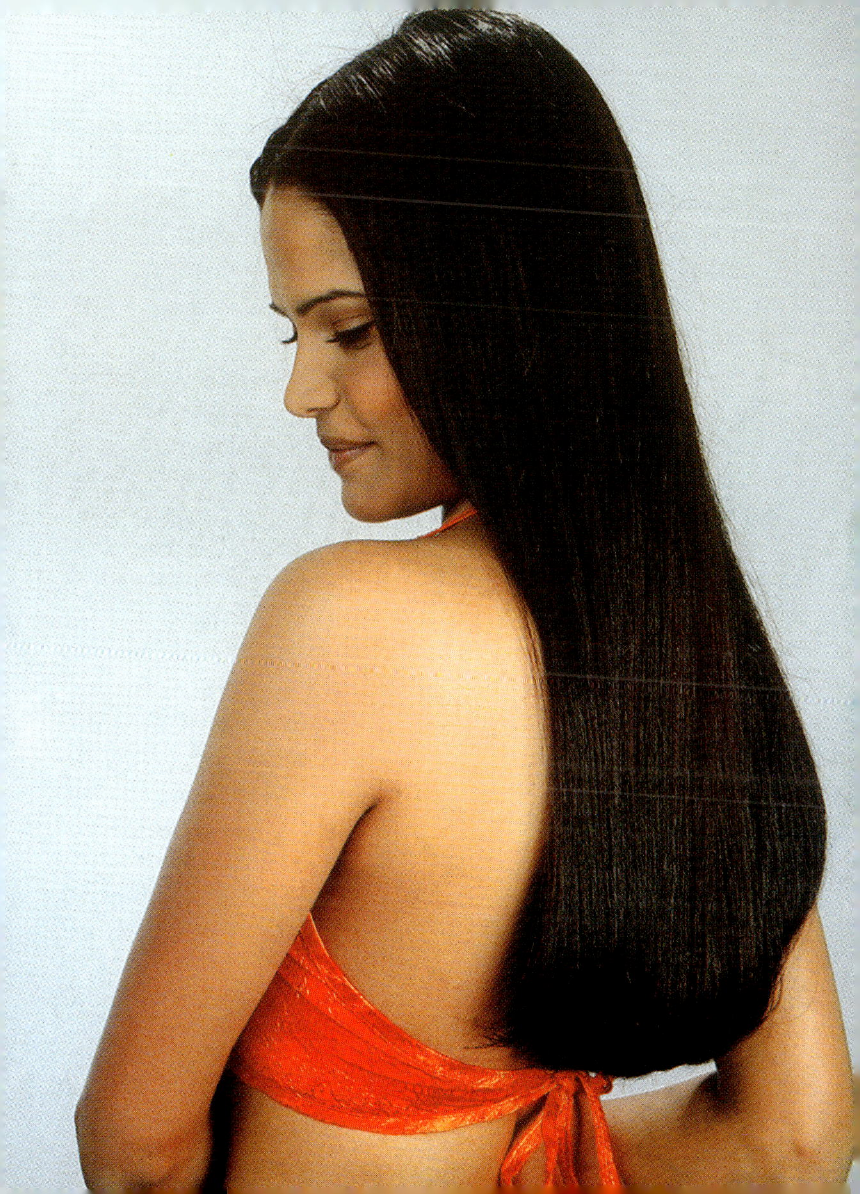

vitalize and purify the bloodstream. The easy way out? Eat at least one orange a day. Simple!

Teeth and Bones: These need calcium and Vitamin D. So take plenty of milk and fish. Avoid too much of starch and sugar. This builds healthy and strong teeth and bones.

Hair: Hair is made from a protein-based substance called keratin. Thus, a healthy mane of hair needs plenty of protein and vitamin B. A high protein diet should include fish, cheese and eggs.

Nails: To avoid chipping, cracking and discolouring of nails, ensure that you have a diet rich in proteins and minerals and iodine.

Eyes: The most essential requirement for healthy eyes is Vitamin A. Carrots and cabbage and other leafy vegetables are a good source, as are butter, eggs and fish.

Over the years, our eating habits have deteriorated. Coupled with the fact that pesticides are being used in grains, fruits and vegetables, eventually they rob you of essential "natural"nutrients. Today's working women seek a quick and easy way out. Thus, many people go in for processed foods, which may be the primary cause of poor nutrition. There is really no substitute for nature. We have seen it time and again. Natural produce, fruits, vegetables and food grains are best when grown in its natural process without any artificial ingredients. An increasingly large number of people are depriving themselves of essential nutrients. True, the modern, stressful lifestyle may be a cause, but lack of interest and ignorance about the basic nutritional values is definitely the other cause.

In today's lifestyle, busy people with little time for shopping for food and even lesser time for cooking it, do not realise the harmful effects of only relying on processed foods. Besides, the marketing hype and fashion cults often change, dictate and shape people's food habits. Be wary of such sensationalism. Do not become a prey to these superficial swings in food habits, for they are based on economics and your health is never the consideration. A bit of intuitive know how and a lot of commonsense can steer you to a healthy way of eating for a more beautiful you.

One of the most glaring bad food habits that exist today is subsistence on hastily prepared foods or convenience foods as they are called. These are semi-processed add-some-water-type of preparations. Thus, essential minerals are robbed from your food. Today's staple diet consists of foods that are used as snacks. Lack of time, or rather the lack of priority in one's life are the reasons why one so often picks up bad eating habits. If you plan ahead, and educate yourself about the nutritive values of common day-to-day food products, you can eat well and grow beautiful. Let your body "talk" about the food it needs.

There is also a need to dispel some myths about food, nutrients and diet. Some believe that the key to health and beauty is by increasing the daily dose of vitamins. So popping pills becomes a common everyday occurrence. You may not even need to take pills unless you are short on any particular vitamin that you may need to supplement. Mindless pill popping is harmful. Excess is worse than deficiency.

Your Kitchen
A Treasure Trove

Nature has been very generous with its bounty of fruits, flowers, vegetables and herbs. It gives us all that we need to look beautiful, remain healthy and stay youthful.

Plants have provided man with his total needs. Foods that sustain us and help us to remain healthy. Vitamins and minerals that meet the total needs of the body. Fruits, vegetables and herbs that give a special sparkle to the eyes; luster to the hair and colour to the cheeks.

The early Egyptians were the first to take an interest in using plants for making perfumes and cosmetics. They perhaps learnt the art from the Mesolithic travellers who roamed the Nile valley in 5,000 to10,000 BC.

The Egyptians had a cure and a preparation for every part of the body. Ancient Egyptian women improved and enhanced their appearances with a variety of cosmetics made from the Earth's bounty.

A judicious use of nature's gifts helps you to enhance your assets and improve upon your drawbacks. It certainly makes you aware that beauty and health are intertwined. Good nutrition and use of natural beauty aids can radiate that aura of beauty that was dormant within you. With the use of these fruits, vegetables, flowers and herbs, you can improve the quality of your hair, texture of your skin and in fact rejuvenate yourself completely.

Health and confidence will reflect not only on your face but also in your complete personality. So, go ahead and make yourself beautiful, not by putting layers of make-up but by enhancing the quality of your skin; hair, and complexion. And by, being content and happy with the way you look naturally. Be beautiful and happy from within.

We owe it to ourselves to spend a little time and effort to grow beautiful. Equipped with these helpful hints from skincare; hair care, face care to nutritional guidelines, you can discover ways to improve your looks and remain youthful and beautiful.

Before you decide on a course of self-improvement, you first need to do a thorough body-check. Recognize your weak beauty points and set about the task of improving upon them and enhancing them. Every product cannot give you a miraculous cure. Using products to improve and enhance yourself has to be a determined and deliberate effort, and it has to fit into a normal routine of your lifestyle. Decide what is best for you; what enhancers you really need and then go about using them regularly to show results and maintain them.

When you are young, you have enough time and spare cash to look after yourself. But as you take on responsibilities of home, hearth and children, beauty care need not take a back seat for want of time or money, if you use the products so easily available in your own kitchen.

Today, beauty houses the world over are being compelled to go back to nature; to use more natural products in their preparations. The modern woman is going back to nature, both in her eating habits and for her body care. Homemade natural beauty aids can prove to be effective if used correctly and consistently.

As you would have realized after going through the beauty care suggestions; fruits, flowers, herbs and vegetables provide cures for improving the quality of the skin, giving a glow to a tired face, imparting health, colour and body to your hair, thus imparting a sense of well-being to the complete body. True, these beauty cures do not have a shelf life, as they contain no preservatives or chemicals. However, you just need to analyse what you need to use everyday, or every week. Once you establish a routine, the task of making and using them is worth the effort of making them fresh. So, spare a little time for yourself.

Let us now take a look at what your beauty treasure trove in the kitchen has to offer. Indeed your kitchen is like an eco-friendly cosmetic laboratory. It provides you with beauty aids for almost every problem and helps you to overcome flaws, if any, and to enhance your beauty. These cures usually have no side effects and instead beautify you from within and not merely superficially.

Let us now recapitulate some of the most easily available beauty cure aids available right here in your kitchen:

ALMOND: The juice of Almonds, crushed and powdered almonds are extensively used to make face packs, skin nourishers and night creams that nourish and 'feed' your skin. They are extremely useful on aged or wrinkled skins. Usually mixed with rose water and glycerin to make skin nourishers. When added to milk, makes an excellent mask that nourishes and softens your skin.

APPLE: Apple juice if mixed with Vinegar makes an excellent hair rinse. Grated apple paste mixed with honey or milk makes an excellent facemask, very useful for complexion cures.

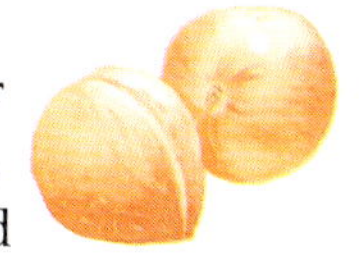

APRICOT: Fresh apricots blended with honey or milk; or fresh apricot paste by itself makes excellent face-masks, which is a very effective nourisher for dry skin, chapped arms, and it helps in rejuvenating dead skin.

AVOCADO: This is a universal favourite. The pulp of this fruit is a skin nourisher and provides an excellent 'food' for the skin. If added to honey or curds, it makes an excellent moisturizer.

BANANA: Pulp if mixed with milk, honey or curds makes a good face-mask that rids you of blemishes. An excellent skin softener. Pulp when mixed with curd and beaten to a thick paste is excellent for your hair, promotes healthy, glossy hair and gives them a unique shine.

CARROT: The ideal 'wrinkle fighter'. Raw carrots grated and added to almond oil and honey and applied as a thick mask, fights wrinkles.

CHICKPEA POWDER: Used as a base for different types of face-masks and as a skin softener and exfoliate. It helps to remove dead skin; hair on the arms and blemishes as well as acne.

COCONUT OIL: Used in numerous beauty care aids. Excellent hair nourisher.

CUCUMBER: Some of the best skin preparations are made from cucumber. When used with curds, makes good, nourishing complexion masks. When used by itself, its juices remove dark circles and blemishes. An excellent skin tauter; it also closes pores, fights skin tan and helps in rejuvenating the skin.

GARLIC: Good for its medicinal properties. If taken raw, it purifies the blood, thus giving a clearer complexion. It also heals cuts and wounds, and clears blemishes if its juice is applied.

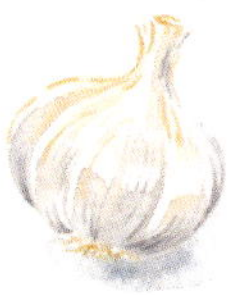

GRAPEFRUIT: When the fruit is blended with yogurt it makes a good skin tonic. A skin tautner that also cures blemishes and shadows.

HONEY: A pre-requisite for so many skin nourishers; face-masks and skin tonics. If taken daily with lime and warm water, it purifies blood and clears the skin of blemishes.

HENNA: Its leaves are dried and powdered. Used not only to decorate and beautify the palms, it is universally used as a hair conditioner, colorant and nourisher.

LAVENDER: Its flowers are used to make soaps and hair creams. the oils in these flowers promote hair growth. You can make excellent toilet waters from it to soothe tired nerves. Its essential oils are excellent coolants for headaches and migraines.

LEMON: One of the most commonly used ingredients. A perfect all-rounder used for removing skin tans; as a facemask; as an astringent, as a skin toner and lightener. It tautens the skin and removes wrinkles. Useful to fight dandruff and an excellent tonic if imbibed with honey.

LILAC: Its flowers not only yield a wonderful perfume, they make excellent astringents, bath waters, and soothe sunburnt skin.

MARIGOLD: Its flowers are used to make face creams and skin ointments. It is soothing to the eyes too.

ONION: Onion juice can again be used in various beauty cure treatments. Its juice cures pimples, burn scars and is excellent for dandruff problems. It also helps to restore natural hair colour.

OATS: An excellent base for making face packs, exfoliates and is a remarkable skin tightener.

OLIVE: Used to prepare skin creams to nourish the skin. Revives jaded skin and good for dull, lifeless hair.

PAPAYA: Again, an excellent and commonly used base for face packs and an excellent hair conditioner. It adds bounce and shine to the hair. The papaya is easily available and its regular use does wonders for your skin and hair.

PEACH: An all time favourite with beauticians all over the world. Makes nourishing facemasks and packs. Fights dry skin and curbs wrinkles. Exfoliates and nourishes.

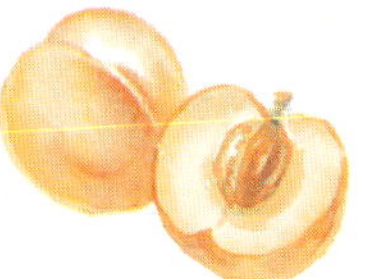

POTATO: A remarkable skin tautner and helps lighten tan. Heals burns, cuts and lightens your complexion. Helps to get rid of burn marks, removes pimples and freckles.

ROSE: Its petals are used to make a number of beauty preparations and astringents. It softens the skin, fights dry chapped skin and soothes jaded skin.

SAFFRON: Skin enhancer and softener. Excellent for the complexion.

SAGE: Used as a hair colorant. If used with olive oil it also nourishes dry, lifeless hair.

SANDALWOOD: Commonly associated with making perfumes. Its powder when mixed with honey or milk enhances the skin miraculously. It fights tanning; softens the skin and is an excellent cure for pimples, blackheads and blemishes.

STRAWBERRY: Its fruit is crushed and used with milk or honey to make facemasks. Just strawberry juice by itself is an ideal cure for clearing blemishes.

SUNFLOWER: This is also used to cure blemishes.

TUMERIC: Has tremendous curative powers. Cures scars and burn marks. It smoothens the skin and is a base for many other tonics.

TOMATO: Another favourite 'skin toner'. Makes good facemasks. A good cleanser and useful for clearing the skin of marks and blemishes.

WALNUT: Both the fruit and its shell are used to darken the hair. Oils extracted from these are used as hair darkeners and mixed with shampoo to give a sheen and gloss and volume to the hair.

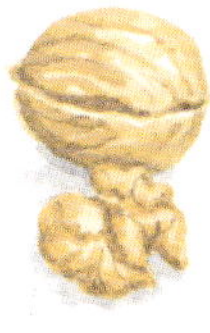

WATERCRESS: Used to clear the skin. It smoothens the skin. A paste made from this when applied on burn marks clears them quickly. A good skin hydrator.

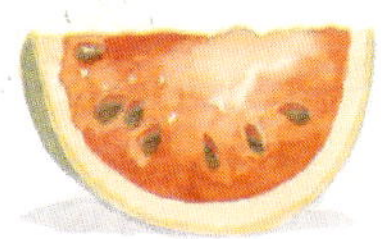

WATERMELON: An ideal skin hydrator. It makes the skin taut, refreshed and rehydrated. It also helps to clear shadows under the eyes. There is no better moisturizer than watermelon.

WHEAT: Its husk, or porridge are good exfoliates. Also used as a base in a number of skin mask preparations.

LETTUCE: Makes an excellent astringent. Fights acne and blemishes.

YOGURT: Used in numerous skin preparations to make skincare masks, packs, and by itself as a skin smoothener. Fights acne. Yogurt is also used in a number of hair care preparations. It nourishes the hair, helping in healthy hair growth.

The magical beauty treasure chest in your own kitchen can help you create your own beauty kit. You can remain beautiful and healthy by using these natural beauty aids. Ultimately, we do fall back on nature to help us become truly beautiful. So give yourself a natural makeover from your own kitchen beauty box, which is indeed a treasure trove of beauty aids.